Rediscovery Journey of a Corporate Persona

Shefali Bansal

CONTENTS

Foreword

A note on the book

Acknowledgements

Index

- SECTION 1: State of affairs when I started my journey
- SECTION 2: Improving physical well-being
- SECTION 3: Improving mental well-being
- SECTION 4: Improving emotional well-being
- SECTION 5: WoW ! I moved my weight
- Interview with my yoga trainer
- About the author

FOREWORD

This book is a culmination of 2 years of rediscovery journey of Shefali Bansal who has been one of my students. This endeavour aims at identifying genuine challenges that one goes through to achieve the happiness journey. It captures how through discipline, focus and guidance, one can achieve the goals while continuing the corporate life

In conclusion, this book is not academic in style or content; its deeply insightful and strongly practical. It aims to instil a constructive confidence among the readers and hopes to inspire many to a healthy lifestyle.

It is not restricted for corporate people alone but for everyone who want to embrace aspects of physical, mental and emotional well-being. I hope many of you can relate to these.

I am happy to see the book been brought to life by Shefali whose capacity to pull out invisible but powerful insights is unparalleled. And when combined with her flair for writing, the result is compelling!

It is rare to see a corporate person at her level to have humbleness & openness to learn and undertake this journey towards wellness. It was rough and challenging for her. I was happy to see her evolution to the path which I would relate to a blossoming of a flower which just needed a catalyst. It was indeed a great experience for me to witness my protégé's journey path.

I wish her the best with my favourite quote 'Just enjoy the path and universe has so much to offer us'

Radha Srinivasan
Soul Listener, Yoga Proponent, A student for Life !

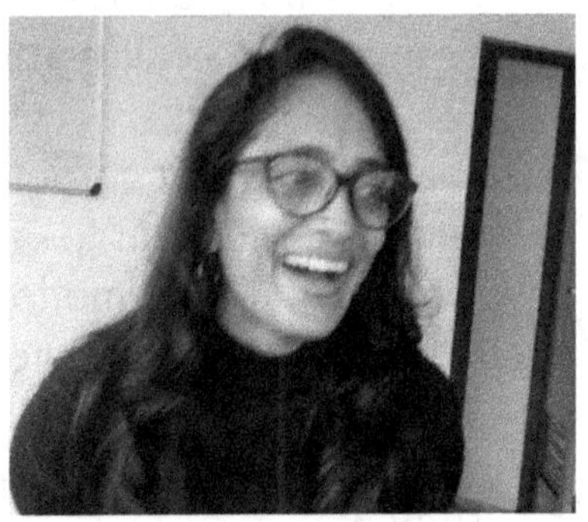

A NOTE ON THE BOOK

My focus while writing this journey book was to inspire folks who are finding themselves trapped in corporate rat race and are unable to focus on their health and well-being.

Through this book, which has been my personal journey over a period of 2 plus years, my endeavour is to provide hope that one can be in corporate world and yet find a work life balance and achieve happiness & healthy body and spirit.

The book has been divided into five sections which essentially were different phases of my rediscovery journey. The book starts with overview of my physical and mental state of affairs when I started my journey about 2 years back. I then talk about the interventions I incorporated to improve my physical, mental and emotional well-being working with my trainer. And finally, I conclude by talking about how this new-found balance (physical, mental, emotional) worked to make the weight loss program a reality.

The book would not have been complete if I did not cover the nuggets of wisdom from my trainer who played crucial role in this journey of mine. This I cover in section titled "Interview with my yoga trainer".

The book is written in a free-flowing style and I hope readers can relate to the examples shared in the book; and find inspiration to take their own Rediscovery journey.

ACKNOWLEDGMENTS

I probably have always skipped this section whenever I read a book. Its only now after writing my first book that I realise how much one truly depends on the work and support of others. It's never ever a solitary effort, even if the name on the title page stands alone.

This book would not have been possible without small army of people.

Thanks to the unshaken support of my husband Rajiv who was rock solid behind my endeavour. He supported me in all ways not just in writing of this book but throughout my rediscovery journey. He took care of all the logistics needed for publishing this book.

Ah…and my children Shubham and Khushi, who provided supported me and kept me motivated when the weighing machine, the mental peace & happiness quotients were not so friendly during the rediscovery journey. They also supported me by displaying adaptability during my fitness journey accommodating to my timings and tantrums.

I owe the whole conceptualisation and initiation of this book to Ms. Radha Srinivasan who is my yoga trainer. She played critical role in providing valuable inputs during the writing of the book. Besides being consistent and passionate crusader for the cause of happiness and health, helped identify nuances which would benefit the audience.

My heartfelt thanks for playing a key role in my rediscovery journey goes to my yoga group where it all started. The friendly, fun filled group was instrumental for my sustenance, motivation & continuation in this wellbeing journey.

A large part of credit for doing critical reviews and providing valuable insights goes to my friends Ms. Ananta Kothari & Ms. Monica Aggarwal. Their openness, helpful hints and ideas on the flow and content of the book were invaluable.

1
STATE OF AFFAIRS WHEN I STARTED MY JOURNEY

How was I in July 2016?

My physical state

- Personally, found myself to be quite low on my physical fitness levels

- Completely sedentary lifestyle would go out of breath even after climbing a single flight of stairs

- Overweight, feeling of tiredness after small chores

- Lethargy-ness, even walking for small distance seemed a tiresome journey

- Long hours at work, followed by evening office calls from home

- Frequent requirement for medication for headache and back pain

- Driving "To & fro" from office seemed tiring

- Lack of sound sleep

- "Not so" healthy eating habits

My mental and emotional state

- Edgy, uneasy, losing patience easily

- Stressed and anxious at most times

- Life toggling between home and work

- Negligible social interactions with friends & relatives

- Questions like what am I trying to achieve? am I happy? which direction is life moving into? started to pop up in my head

At surface level, all looked well and moving on as expected. Someone looking from outside, will see everything going well, good job, kids doing well, happy family.
But internally I knew, something needed to change to bring in changes to my state of affairs.

This led me to dig deeper and do introspection to identify what was the most important things requiring attention.
Physical fitness & my weight management clearly came out as the top areas requiring an attention.

This was July of 2016. And what is destined
to happen does indeed happen.
I accidentally bump into a friend who was
coming from yoga class on a Saturday. It
was life changing meeting for sure. This
chanced meeting happened at a time when I
was looking to adopt a routine / activity
which would help me to improve physical
fitness levels. I decided to give it a try for
this weekend yoga class which my friend
recommended. This was my first time into
the world of yoga!

My inception into Yoga!

-   I started on this weekend yoga class. The
    timing worked well as it did not interfere
    in my weekday corporate work schedule.
    Though, internally I was not sure how
    this new experiment will turn out.

-   My previous experiences on different
    programs for weight loss like dieting,
    physical exercise routines like walking,
    gym over last few years were not much
    success as I used to give up mid-way due
    to lack of instant results.

-   There was something in the yoga class
    that on the very first day I felt at ease. As
    few classes progressed I started to feel

comfortable. I was still figuring out, if it was the fun element I got in the yoga class or the yoga group friendly dynamics or the yoga trainer was the reason.

- The good part here was that, I was regular to the classes for initial few weeks. I also started to earnestly look forward to the weekend class. This was unlike my previous experiments with various classes in the past where I had to motivate myself to continue the classes.

- I found my yoga trainer to be extremely sensitive as I could gather from my interactions in the yoga classes. Once, I was comfortable in the yoga class & the initial honeymoon period over, I took courage to discuss on my physical, mental challenges with my yoga trainer. She was very receptive to these conversations and was equally engaged to help me out. These conversations which were candid; were stepping stone for my journey to improve my physical fitness.

Starting steps

- In the beginning, to start improving my physical fitness, my trainer recommended the following simple goal:

    o Daily 30 minutes yoga asanas in the morning at home

    o The expectation was to have discipline to have this 30-minute morning routine for at least 5-6 days in a week.

The 30 minutes yoga regime*

- This morning routine was suggested by the trainer considering my body weight and muscle flexibility. The routine was combination of asanas which helped in improving the body metabolism, muscle strengthening, toning and flexibility.

- The above routine was peppered with very important breathing exercises.

- If cardio based asanas were like staple rice, the combination of these asanas with breathing & muscle toning exercise provided the required spice to this rice . This made the whole exercise combination healthy and tasty!

My experiences with the 30 minutes regime

- I started doing daily yoga asanas at home in the morning during the week days religiously. There was something magical in the recommendations or my will power or my respect for my trainer that my morning yoga routine was very regular. For most weeks, I could adhere to this routine for 5-6 days in the week.

- This was a significant change from my previous trials on exercise routines. Here I was not only regular in my routine , I was waking quite early every day at 5:30 am and still enjoying. The body itself tuned up for an early morning wake up.

- One of the asanas which did help me was the Surya Namaskar (sun salutation) which is empirically proven asana to provide flexibility to ones' core.

- As a reflect back, these 30 minutes routine created a morning discipline for me. The body started to look forward to doing the asanas every day. At times when I skipped for a day, the internal voice would make me guilty and I would hate to miss any day of my exercise . It started to become a habit. The days where I had to miss the routine owing to kids or factors beyond my control, I would be conscious to get the routine completed in the evening.

Things started to change at physical level

- As body started to get into the asana's routine, I could start seeing improvements on my physical well-being & flexibility of the body in couple of weeks.

- I could start doing certain asanas like Utkatasan, Trikonasana, Bhujangasana, Setubandhan asanas with lot of ease and also could try new variations in these asanas.

While it was satisfying to start seeing the improvements on physical fitness levels through initiation into yoga. I had taken baby steps till now and knew that more needs to be done to improve physical fitness substantially. And "what I did to achieve it", I walk you through in the next section on "Improving physical well-being"

* The readers should consult with a professional trainer before starting any of the regime as the above routine worked for me. It would be different for different people.

2
IMPROVING PHYSICAL WELL-BEING

In a sound body rests a sound mind. Treat your body like temple and consider them sacred if we hope to live life fully.
Every hour exercise adds 3 hours to individual lives. The act of caring for my physical temple reminded me that life greatest pleasures are often life's simplest ones.

As I was starting to become discipline on my daily 30 minutes yoga, I started to see slow improvements happening at my physical fitness levels.
I could start to feel more energetic during the day, the amount of medications I used to require started to come down. I felt less lethargic, the drive to office was not that tiring after all.

I used to feel uneasy the day I used to miss my morning 30 minutes routine due to being under the weather or lack of time due to pressing need on that day.

Owing to this uneasiness which used to linger if I used to skip my routine, I started to give a try to complete my regime on days when I was little under the weather. And magically, I used to find myself a lot better at the end of the routine. I realised it was all a mental block and body is lot more adaptable

One example I would like to quote on how I restarted playing badminton after overcoming my mental block.
I always loved playing badminton, however was unable to do so for last many years due to my knee issue and I always had mental block that I can never play it back. As my physical fitness was improving, I realised I can give a shot at Badminton for 15 minutes for starts. And **wow** I could play back after many years!

Enhanced fitness regime (Morning & Evening)

After seeing my disciplined morning 30 minutes regime and my body's settling down in a flexible mode, my trainer realised that I was ready to increase my fitness regime. The evening routine of my Badminton also gave her motivation to increase my fitness routine in the evening.

She suggested me to start on a 30 minutes fitness regime in the evening's also. This was in addition to my ongoing morning 30 minutes asanas regime.

We did chalk out regime of cardio for the evening for 30 minutes. Considering my health, fitness levels, she suggested cardio exercises like walk, static cycling etc. for the evening regime. With this my evening fitness regime started.

Challenges to overcome for the evening fitness regime

While my morning regime continued on, initially, it was difficult to find time for the evening regime as I had to attend to the evening office calls. Besides the calls, the time for kids, the dinner etc., had to be managed as well.
It took some time and few months for me to get into regime for my evening fitness, but "Wow" it did happen.

I had to move meetings out to start little late in the evening, few I had to delegate and sometimes move my routine to have the exercises late in the evening after the calls, before dinner etc. My family also adjusted to have early dinner which is always advisable.

This also gave me flexibility to perform by evening regime.

My persistence to find solution to the challenges to squeeze these 30 minutes of time for the evening regime helped. Where there is a will, there is a way!.

Learning and experiences on enhanced fitness regime

One of my learnings here was to **Not to Overdo** things.
I used to love playing badminton when I got a chance, and often in flow of things I would over do more than what my knee or body can take. This would result in painful knees. As expected my trainer would not be happy. I started to bring here mental toughness to limit my routine to a level that body can take it. Stop before things break.

I was happy to learn the art of mindful walking. Its walking from being "mind" full to mindful walking. I used to walk for 30 minutes and feel like having done my regime of the day. However, after having done this the routine for many days and seeing much of an impact, I had conversation with my trainer. She asked me to do "mindful" walking. The trainer helped me to put on my head phones with peppy music while walking to avoid the 'mind full' thoughts. This recommendation helped me to start seeing a difference on my fitness.

One of the add on experience which was very important was that I started to become careful on what I was feeding my body. The mind will think twice on what I will eat because I did no wanted to now burn these additional extra calories through exercise. I would rather than avoid them. I did not go for any diet plans but ate home-made food and avoided fried, sweet and high calorie items. Kept the body hydrated and often had warm water. When required to eat outside, I was conscious of what I ate.

The outcome & impact

The morning & evening physical fitness routine started to show outcomes. I could see inch loss happening, I could start to feel young , energetic, agile and most importantly started to feel light and fit.

The evening walk helped me to connect with the community folks who were never aware of my presence. The evening office call management made me prioritise on essentials over the non-essentials. The time which got freed up due to some of the delegated calls, helped the delegates to feel more empowered. It also helped me to utilise this time for more strategic thinking.

My exercise regime was so smooth and doable where I used only my body weight to bring the desirable changes . It also started to show effects on my mental and physiological fitness in couple of months. And my rediscovery of my mental health thru physical health was an eye-opening experience. It's is like an ice breaker to understand that if I give an hour to treat my body, it gives back to me strength from rest of 23 hours including the quality of sleep.

After having fed enough to my physical well-being, my other aspect of mental was asking for more. So, what's mental well-being ?

3
IMPROVING MENTAL WELL-BEING

Corporate life has become a synonym any mental stress just for the fact that it is demanding . Target, time bound, reviews, assessment, evaluation are those which bring the experience of somatisation rather than bringing contentment, joy and passion. The above said sadly make one to forget "being in the zone" whether it's a process , success or any kind of achievement. Corporate community if compulsorily tuned to "what's up next attitude. So, the outcome is "psychosomatic issues " like weight, blood pressure, early diabetics, issues with digestive system, endocrine issues, sleeping issues and many more.

While physical fitness helped in making the body energetic which in turn helped to start bringing focus back on what's essential.

The mind is a monkey as we know and often the most difficult to manage and control. While physical fitness was improving, I often found myself not at ease owing to stresses induced by corporate challenges. And often my mental state was uneasy due to the following factors:

- Over engineering of thoughts
- "What If" thoughts
- Stress
- Fear of Failure
- Anxieties
- Long hours at work including weekends
- People's perceptions
- "What next" syndrome
- Lack of sleep

And I realized the above needed to be taken care to feel strong physically and mentally.

I did have deep discussion with my trainer who is also trained therapist in this area. And there were wonderful suggestions which came from her, which I started to incorporate.

These were everyday suggestions and most of you can relate to it. The key point was to really bring these into execution.

- Breathing & Meditation
- Looking at fears and anxieties in objective manner
- Time boxing the office work

☐ Applying corporate nuggets of wisdom

I am happy to share my experiences when I adopted the above suggestions made by my trainer.

Breathing & Meditation

Breathing is very intrinsic part of yoga, however to really get benefitted from deep breathing, it's important to imbibe principles of pranayama. I like everyone believed I was doing breathing. We all breathe as we are all alive. However, it was all about mindful breathing. My trainer who loves to make "People Breathe" was no forgiving when she was categorical to say that you are not breathing. She helped to explain the fundamentals of deep, long mindful breathing. Was it easy for me to do mindful breathing? The answer is "No" and I share my personal experience with the breathing exercises and I am sure this will resonate with most corporate folks.

- Sitting at-least for 10 full minutes just for breathing is extremely challenging
- One finds time for everything else except for true breathing
- 10 minutes sitting for breathing looks quite long and one thinks of completing

two office meetings in the time frame
than to sit for breathing

- As one finally accepts and starts to adopt breathing, a lot of questions come up on breathing duration (is 5 minutes breathing not sufficient over 10 minutes?), style, depth etc.
- Slowly with daily practice, one starts to settle down for 10 minutes breathing with support. The support here are the tools that helps mind remaining in present. For everyone different techniques work, for me listening to soulful music along with breathing worked.
- Our time, as one becomes comfortable, the aim should be to extend the breathing which helps in calming of the mind and thereby helps in connecting to the internal soul
- It took me time to reach to a stage where I could sit for 10 minutes breathing / pranayama. I am on my way in experiencing the true essence of breathing as a corporate person as breathing indeed helps to relieve mental stress.

Meditation is a big topic and I do think I am still a beginner on it. My journey on this has just started and by the time I complete this book, I would be better in experiencing the benefits of it and would look to cover my experiences in my next book ☺.

Looking at fears and anxieties in objective manner

This was an important one as often in corporate mad race, one forgets to look at issues in objective manner. The fear of failure often clouds the judgement. One of the change which I incorporated was to start looking at fears, anxieties, challenges in very objective way. This was often done by stepping back and looking at issues from different perspective. I realized often most of the anxieties cropped up because of our over-analysis or over-engineering thoughts. Discussion with colleagues, friends and family on sticky issues helped me bring in fresh thought process or an objective viewpoint.

Time boxing the office work

My office hours were long which were not allowing me to get mental break. I was working 7 days a week including the weekend. I started looking at mechanisms on how I can start to time box the amount of time spent at office work. This was a major change I had to adopt as for a workaholic like me it was always difficult.

But I persisted and knew that I had to make this happen. Some of the changes which I adopted:
- Stopped working over weekends (Saturday & Sunday) for the office work
- Minimal office work over Sunday (off course exceptions were there for customer critical situations which were supported as required)
- Critical prioritization of work-related requirements (do, delegate, delay)
- Starting the day early but winding up the evening calls & work by 10:00 pm in the night.
- Quick decision making also helped to avoid backlog of pending works
- Extreme high focus on essentials over non-essentials at home & office also helped in channelizing the energy in right areas

Initially the above was tough but over period of time, body and mind started getting used to this routine. I was super happy to see that this helped me to start getting adequate sleep in the night as well!

Applying corporate Nuggets of wisdom

Based on my conversation with my trainer, I started to apply nuggets of wisdom for corporate world which helped me in improving my mental wellbeing. The focus started to slowly move towards working smart than just working hard.

- The external forces should not change your unique nature.
- Read every day something new & keep building skills (When one learns something new, its empirically proven that brain expands and human's feel happy)
- Don't be hard & harsh on yourself
- Do we need to be perfect all the time?
- It's not because things are difficult that we do not dare, it's because we don't dare that they become difficult
- Don't worry about things you can't change
- Enjoy the path more than focusing on reaching the destination
- Respond and not react

Impact & outcome

The incorporation of the above activities in my lifestyle started to help me provide clarity of thoughts. I could find myself to be quite relaxed at most times and could see myself more outgoing and coming out of a cocoon. As I started to apply the above nuggets and make progress, I was happy to see my mental toughness and well-being improving. As my

physical and mental wellness started to happen,
I could see my emotional wellness started to
improve as well.

In my mind I was still looking for taking my
happiness & emotional well-being quotient to
next level. And how did I eventually get there?,
I talk more about it in the next section on
"Emotional Well-being"

4
IMPROVING EMOTIONAL WELL-BEING

The body and mind wellness would not have been complete without emotional wellbeing. It's all about mind, body and soul. The soul's enrichment is an important element and when this taken care of, it plays an important role for person's happiness.

And I could sense that while things started to become better for me physically and mentally, somewhere I was not having this inner feeling of happiness.

This was an important area where I had deep discussions with my trainer. Her recommendations were very simple. These simple recommendations often get forgotten somewhere in corporate rate race.

I am covering some of the recommendations which my trainer suggested here:

☐   Do what your heart wants

☐   Enjoy the small things in life
☐   Understand the difference between love and attachment as often most unhappiness occurs due to attachment

Candidly, it was difficult for me to adopt the recommendations as long corporate life had created so many artificial layers that I had forgotten on what gave me happiness, what made my heart sing with joy. A lot of the recommendations required me to virtually go back in time. It required me to start un-layering a lot of mental layers which were created over years in corporate life. It was not easy at all but if one persists, this is doable and achievable.

I share below **my experiences** as I adopted the above recommendations of my trainer for improving mental well-being

Do what your heart wants
I was in this world where keep running sprints to win the Olympic gold. I started realizing this was a myth when I started considering my office and work life pattern. I was only living in two worlds of office and home. In these two worlds, my strong assumption was that, I never had time for myself or time to enjoy small moments & joys. For me, it was "Soleful" state instead of "Soulful" state.

In this journey of finding my soul, it was extremely difficult to even identify bucket list of things which my heart wanted to do.
Working with my trainer and going back in time and identifying things which made me happy in the past, I was finally able to come up with my happiness list.
With one major step achieved, my trainer suggested to focus on picking 2-3 things at a time and executing on them than to boil the ocean. After all, the intent was to run the marathon of life and have inner sense of happiness.
As I start to execute and complete the selected activities, I started to take on newer set of activities from the list and keep making progress. And within a year, I did a lot of things which I always wanted to do but had no time due to corporate layering.

My experiences when I followed my heart and the bucket list of things I accomplished

- I started enjoying the journey than the destination most of the time (I am still learning ☺)
- Connected back with friends and relatives at more personal level than social media level

- Finding time for kids for their special occasions like PTM, Sports day, annual day celebrations
- Exploration and experiential learning on few hobbies which I always wanted to do but had taken back burner
- Started contributing to the volunteering activity (feed Bangalore campaign)
- Trying new musical instrument like Dholak
- Playing again my favorite sport badminton & table tennis
- Clothing style - Sarees were slowly coming back for special occasions.
- Writing is back in vogue - Blog writing, book writing
- Local community connect – I started to know folks beyond my neighbors.
- Book Reading was back - finished reading of lot of technical, autobiography books
- Experimenting with new stuff- I started to try my hand on singing which my heart always wanted to do. It was a nervy start, but I am getting comfortable as I pen this. Keep listening to your heart!
- Dabbled for few weeks to learn dancing. It did not go very far but happy to have given a try.

- Travelling to hometown after many years to meet up with my old friends and relatives. These trips were so much soul satisfying.
- Connecting with school alumni and school friends
- Travelling out impromptu with friends, kids without much planning
- Speaking at external event for the company. Started as a shy nervous speaker to a speaker who could speak on various technology, client topics
- Watching movie in theatre with family after many years
- Doing more mentoring and coaching sessions at the workplace which I always loved
- **Letting your hair down** is an important factor that plays such a vital role in improving one's happiness. In this context I wanted to quote my experience with my friendly yoga group that provided me this platform to let my hair down. With my crazy friendly yoga group, I had fun along with yoga learnings. It helped me to be myself. In the group, I was not representing any company, it was just me. The fun and frolic we had during the yoga sessions provided moments for your heart to sing. The corporate world sometimes makes

you to act, react and behave in certain ways, here there was no such barriers. We enjoyed our small girl/ladies talks, try out crazy ideas during birthday celebrations. I celebrated my last birthday with the theme of "bring forward the child in you ".

My learning from the above experience were:
- Loving yourself is very important for one's happiness.
- Remain yourself.
- No comparisons.
- Non-judgmental.
- Play on your strengths.

Enjoy the small things in life

One of the other suggestion my trainer had to improve mental well-being was to start enjoying small things in life. Often in the corporate world we are sucked into this unending timelines and pressures that we forgot to observe small and beautiful things happening around us. We forget to appreciate that Universe has so much to offer but we fail to do so as we are either worrying about future or the past events which have happened.

To really enjoy small things, it's important we stay in present. It took me a while to enjoy small things in life. **Sharing here few of my experiences as I adopted this approach:**

- Vasudhaiva Kutumbakam – I started looking at each individual bringing in unique perspective, knowledge and value to the world. This helped to broaden my circle of friends and colleagues & well-wishers. It also started to keep me well-grounded and humble in my interactions with all.
- I started to observe beauty around me (things, humans, nature). The observations helped me to appreciate the uniqueness, talent, wealth of knowledge that universe offers us.
- Earlier I would look at presence of certain people and things to make me happy. Now I did not need it.
- I started finding happiness in small daily interactions like when I provided a helping hand, even in small chores like getting the car parked straight in a small parking slot, even small acts which brought smiles on others brought happiness.
- Simple act of collecting & smelling of flower "Parijat" from which I derived my name was in itself an enriching experience.

- One example I would like to quote to explain this better.
  I was feeling quite homesick during my recent travel to Chicago. This was happening as I was travelling away from family after many days. When I landed, I cleared my mind to stay in present. This helped me to connect and make friends with my new colleagues and I enjoyed my stay thoroughly. I also found a good gym at the hotel which took care of my physical fitness needs. The whole stay in subzero weather at Chicago become enjoyable happened because of my ability to look for small things, adapting to new circumstances with open mind.

I realized as mind, heart starts to open up to the world, you tend to explore more which in turns bring happiness

Understanding the difference between love and attachment

One of the recommendation for emotional well-being from my trainer was to have clarity on difference between love and attachment.

This was a big botheration area for me as I was attached to too many things; attachment with work, attachment with people, attachment with emotions. We often associate attachment with loving someone or something. The two emotions get mixed up which causes sorrow. Hence, it was important to appreciate and understand the differences between the two.

It took lot of interactions with my trainer to understand the difference. We deliberated, debated, had difference of opinion. All I can say it was not easy to say the least. It was a year long journey to start appreciating the value of detachment in small ways. The period was challenging and often stressful.

Once you understand the difference between Love and attachment, I can bet you, your life will be lot meaningful, satisfying and fulfilling. Here is my humble attempt to bring out the differences between the two to help my readers.

Love is *unconditional*
Attachment is *conditional*

Love *bonds* people
Attachment *binds* people

Love is an *experience*
In attachment, we add our *interpretation to the experiences*

Love is step *forward*

Attachment is *step back*

Love is an *inner engineering*
Attachment is *over engineering*

Love creates *effect*
Attachment *affects*

Love wants the *other person to be happy*. If the person reciprocates it's great, but otherwise also it should be immaterial.
Attachment comes with *expectations*.

Love is like *rubber band*
Attachment is like *looped-in*

Love is *liberation*
Attachment is *deliberation*

Love is *being human*
Attachment is *human being*

Love *breaks boundaries*
Attachment *makes boundaries*

The impact and outcome
The understanding of the difference between the two helped me to identify what I truly loved and what all I was attached to. And that it's

important to build the following two attributes to address the challenges of love and attachment:
- Ability to Accept other person's point of view & circumstances
- Let Out & Let Go

Developing an acceptance and let go attitude helped me immensely in my mental well-being. I could understand other's perspectives better. The "Let-go" attitude was very liberating one. It helped me to focus on what I could control and let go of things, aspirations, emotions and people who were not in my control. Unclutter the mind of unwanted baggage. The mind & soul felt lot more contended and happier. The happiness quotient improved significantly.

Though my body, mind and soul were coming together, there was one thing still lingering in my mind "I was still overweight"!
And how did I handle it? Readers let me walk you through my journey as "How I moved my weight"

5
WoW ! I MOVED MY WEIGHT

While I was physically, mentally and emotionally feeling good compared to the time when I started my journey, my body weight was still on a higher side. I was overweight per the BMI scales.

While I was aware of myself being overweight I was happy in my zone and was not really thinking of doing anything aggressively to reduce my body weight. That's where the trainer who has been with you in the journey and who has seen the progress and understands your strengths and challenges becomes so very important.

My trainer realized that it was important that my routine and my body and mind first gets the physical, mental and emotional wellness in place before I start on a weight loss program. When she saw that my body, mind and soul were coming together, she discussed with me on the health risks due to obesity. And suggested if I was ready to start fitness regime which would help me to reduce weight over a period of time.

While I was always knowing that weight loss is required, I was somewhere not convinced if I can do it as all my previous attempts were not successful.

This time it was different. I had someone working very closely with me on the weight loss program. Also, I had spent 1.5 years of disciplined approach on my yoga regime and thus somewhere I had this knack that it's going to work but still was not 100% confident

So here we had deep conversation between me and my trainer on weight loss approach to adopt. I was suggested a tailor-made exercise regime which was roughly two and half times more than what I have been doing regularly. It required me to start my day at 5 am in morning and find way to do minimum 1 hour of exercise in morning and 1 hour in the evening. All looked so unreal considering my unpredictable evening routine due to my office calls. I had struggled earlier to find 30 minutes of time for evening fitness regime. And on top of it, I was given a target weight I should lose at the end of each week. This all sounded so crazy at the start.

I worked with my trainer to define my morning and evening 1-hour regime. Since the focus now was on weight loss, the fitness regime was more on cardio exercises. The 1-hour regime in morning comprised of cardio exercises like Tabata, Cardio asanas like crunches, leg races, planks, sun salutations etc. My evening regime was focused on brisk walk (minimum 30 minutes) followed by stepper or gym cycling. My trainer used to share a weekly schedule for morning, evening regime and I was expected to provide an update in the evening.

This time around during my weight loss program, something magical was happening for sure and I can see cosmic also contributing to make my exercise program a success.

The day I decided to take a shot at it, everything started to fall in place.
I was able to wake up at 5 am and complete my 1 hour of exercise in the mornings. I could figure out to time to find 1 hour to do my evening exercises. If you want something, adjustments are necessary. I adjusted my office calls so that I could find time to exercise. My priority towards health became more important. I also realized that when I take that one hour, the world does not end, work still goes on as usual. Now that I was mentally tough, I got ease out my mind of the main worry that I used to have like people at work will think less of me. I

will be passed over for a promotion. I will not look dedicated enough.

This was so different compared to the time when I just could not figure out way to find any personal time in the evenings. The daily report out on my progress also kept me honest and, on my toes, to make the progress happen. And I could follow my routine for 5-6 days in a week. Rarely a cheat day.

During this routine I became extra conscious on what I was feeding my body. I avoided junk foods, sweets and monitored my eating out. I gave off my daily routine of tea drinking. I did not do dieting, it was all about eating healthy and keeping one adequately hydrated.

And the results:
- I started to lose at healthy 2 kgs. a month. These were my weights which were like sticking with me for so many years
- In about 5 months I lost about 10 kgs. of the weight.
- **The weight scales moved from 87 kg to 74 kg**

Factors contributing to weight loss program

I contribute the weight loss progress to focus, self-discipline on exercise food and constant interaction with my trainer. To sum it up the biggest factors which contributed to it included:
- There is a right time for everything and when the time is right, everything starts to fall in place on its own. The whole ecosystem comes together to make it happen. Mental, physical well-being, environment, all have to come together
- Very important to have a coach and a trainer during the journey who keeps pushing you and motivating you during the "Down" times [Weighing machine does not always gives you good feelings)
- Support of the family as they need to bear with your schedules and down times :)

And the journey continues

Today as I reflect back on my 2 years journey, I have come a long way on my physical, mental and emotional well-being. The changes I can see in my state of affairs include:

-   Full of energy and life
-   Looking forward to taking on more challenges
-   Contended, Happy with mind at ease
-   Found an ability to balance corporate work schedule and still find to keep the soul nourished.

There is still a long way to go for me as there are still more to be done to make the BMI Scores and Mindful scores to be happy. Hence, the journey of learning and continue to build on physical, mental & emotional well-being continues on.

I am hoping my journey inspires you to start your own rediscovery journey. Good luck and best wishes to you all.

Interview with my yoga trainer

My yoga trainer Ms. Radha Srinivasan played key role in my rediscovery journey and hence I do believe the book would only be complete by hearing to her thoughts on health and wellness. Ms. Radha who is a firm believer of *Mastering mind over matter , Universe has so much to offer when you are receptive, make as many people smile when you are alive and make as many cry when you die* has been a yoga trainer for 12 plus years. She has experience of working with hundreds of yoga students spanning across the fraternity of corporate, sports, academia, women & students.

I caught up with Ms. Radha over an interview. Sharing excerpts from this conversation.

As a trainer, how do you address the different needs of the people who approach you?

Everyone's Need is variant. Some come for improving fitness, some for improving flexibility, most for weight loss and some for weight gain too.

Some are already working on some program but are looking for an external push to bring them to their optimum level of fitness.

Yoga is much more than physical level of fitness and everyone wants to adopt it as we are in fast paced era. Hence tangible aspect for oneself is to be physically fit.
Beyond physical level, its mental level, it's an intangible level. This has massive level of impact to individuals but not everyone realises it.

Whoever comes for physical fitness level, I will connect at their level and needs and look to provide a regime which suits their wellbeing.
I would also make them understand that yoga is all about mastering mind over body. Help them to take the journey where they can achieve mind over matter.
Its empirically proven that I can help anyone master one's mind, one can convince thyself and hence convince others.

Why do you think connecting with inner self is important ?

Most of the time, everyone is connecting with external world. This connect may be positive or negative, while chasing behind materialism, success, fame, wealth, leadership etc. We are always connected with external world. And this requires a lot of energy. And at the end we get very little in return compared to what we aspired for and this leads to unhappiness.

What yoga helps to go inwards, understand yourself, it helps you to leverage the energy which is available in abundance within one self. And how do we get this energy? This energy comes from our self-introspection to understand "who we are", "what makes us happy" and similar questions which helps us connect with ourselves.

The moment we understand what makes us happy, we can continue the journey with peace and calm, irrespective of the external influences.
And this is beginning of happiness and it's a journey. It's not a destination and when one starts to understand this, they can see 'how beautiful is the life'.

ABOUT THE AUTHOR

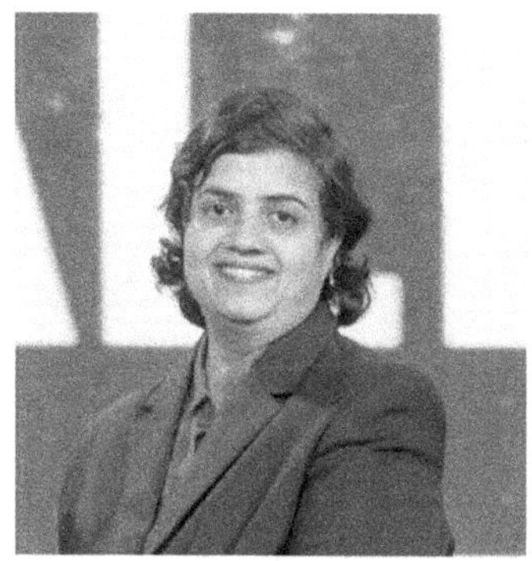

Shefali Bansal is Program Director with IBM India Software Labs.

She is an Engineer with specialisation in Computer Science. A patent holder and winner of numerous recognitions like *Women in Technology, Outstanding Technology Achievement Awards, Best of Analytics* to her credit.

Human performance, taking on challenges and understanding of human behaviours and technology innovations fascinates her. She loves mentoring and spends considerable time for growth of the new generation of technologists. Shefali lives in Bangalore with her husband and 2 kids